Paleo Diet

Paleo Diet Recipes Cookbook

Howard Benson

<u>TERMS & CONDITIONS</u>

No part of this cookbook can be transmitted or reproduced in any form, including electronic, print, photocopying, scanning, recording or mechanical without prior written permission of the author. All information, ideas and guidelines are for educational purpose only. Though the author has tried to ensure the utmost accuracy of content, all readers are advised to follow instructions at their risk. The author of this book cannot be held liable for any incidental damage, personal or commercial caused by misrepresentation of information. Readers are encouraged to seek professional help when needed.

TABLE OF CONTENTS

Chapter 1 – Why Paleo Diet?

Paleo Diet also known as the diet of our ancestors is a powerful diet. Our ancestors didn't have health problems like we face today in our life. The reason for it is because of their diet, Paleo Diet. It has got plenty of benefits, but for now you should it is an extremely powerful diet. So without further delay let's check out these awesome recipes.

Extra ordinary Apple and Sweet Potato Pancakes

Just wondering about a superb, awesome and delicious recipe that it just a treat for your tongue and tummy. Congratz, your wait is over!!

What you need:

- 2 to 3 teaspoons of ground cinnamon (Divided)
- About 3 medium sized sweet potatoes
- 1 granny smith apple
- 2 to 3 tbsps of grass fed butter
- 8 to 9 tbsps of coconut flour
- 1 to 2 tbsp of agave nectar
- 1 to 2 tsp of vanilla essence
- 1 to 2 teaspoon of sea salt
- 6 pastured eggs

- 1 to 2 teaspoon of baking powder
- Coconut oil, as required to fry the pancakes

Procedure:

1. Assemble all the items at one place.
2. Please peel the sweet potato and cut into 1-inch cubes.
3. Peel the apple and chop it finely.
4. Take a skillet and place the grass-fed butter in it along with a tsp of ground cinnamon.
5. Set the flame to medium heat.
6. Cook till butter is totally melted and hot, and then put the chopped apples in it.

7. Cook and whisk until the apples are tender. When the apples are soft, take out and set aside.

8. Now take a large saucepan and fill it with water.

9. Place about 1/2 tsp salt in the water.

10.   Bring the water to a boil.

11.   When the water is boiling, place the sweet potatoes in it.

12.   Boil for 10 to 15 minutes, until the sweet potatoes are tender.

13.   Drain the sweet potatoes and set them apart.

14.   Now take a mixing bowl and put the coconut flour in it along with the sea salt, baking powder and the remaining 1 teaspoon of ground cinnamon. Blend well and set aside.

15. Take a food processor and place the sweet potatoes in it.

16. Run the processor till the potatoes take the form of a puree.

17. Then put the vanilla extract, pastured eggs and agave nectar in the processor.

18. Run the processor again until all the items are well blended.

19. Now put the coconut flour mixture in the processor.

20. Run the processor till the flour is thoroughly mixed with all the other items.

21. Take a griddle or frying pan and place about a teaspoon of oil in it.

22.	When the oil is hot, put about a cup of pancake batter in it.

23.	Fry the pancake above the medium low flame. When one side is brown, toss and brown the other side.

24.	Now for the final step.

25.	Fry all the other pancakes.

26.	Now you can serve the pancakes with the apple-cinnamon mixture.

27.	Enjoy!

Fantasy Banana Walnut Muffins
(three)

So what are you waiting for? The supreme recipe is just below!! Learn it by heart.

What you need:

- ¼ teaspoon Celtic sea salt
- ¼ cup coconut oil
- 1/2 to 1 cup walnuts, toasted and shredded
- 3 dates (Pitted)
- 3 eggs
- 10 drops stevia
- ¼ cup coconut flour
- 2 to 3 medium bananas
- 1/2 to 1 teaspoon baking soda

Procedure:

1. Assemble all the items.
2. Preheat oven to about 350 to 355 F.
3. Place the eggs, dates, bananas, and stevia in a blender and blend at medium speed till blended.
4. Now is the most important step.
5. You should add coconut flour, salt and baking soda, blending until smooth.
6. Fold the walnuts in.
7. One thing remains to be done now.
8. Scoop ¼ cup batter into a muffin pan that is either greased or may be lined.
9. Bake for 20 to 25 minutes, until they're browning and not soft to the touch.

10.	Smell the aroma and serve.

Servings: 9 to 11

Preparation Time: 10 to 15 minutes

Cooking Time: 20 to 25 minutes

Legendary Paleo Pancakes
Prepared with Almond Flour

What you need:

- 2 to 3 tablespoons maple syrup
- Coconut oil, for cooking
- 1 to 2 cup almond flour
- 2 eggs
- 1/3 cup coconut milk
- Sea salt, to taste

Procedure:

1. Assemble all the items.
2. In an expansive blending dish, consolidate the majority of the fixings, away from the coconut oil, and combine well with a wooden spoon — till a player is framed.

3. Over medium warmth, warm the coconut oil in a vast skillet.

4. Drop almost ¼ measure of hitter onto the skillet. Start cooking until air pockets show up on the flapjack surface, or for roughly 2 to 5 minutes.

5. One thing remains to be done now.

6. At the point when air pockets show up, toss the flapjacks with an elastic spatula, and cook for extra 5 to 10 minutes.

7. Top with new berries, nuts, margarine, ghee, whipped coconut cream, stevia, a little cinnamon, crude nectar, and a touch of maple syrup or your other top pick, solid fixings. Now you can serve.

8. Smell the aroma and serve.

Mystical Asparagus with Prosciutto

My mom used to cook this for me. It tastes so amazing. This recipe was a mystic to me till my mom told me how to make it.

What you need:

- 80 to 85 g (1 serving) Prosciutto ham
- 90 to 100 g (6 medium spears) asparagus

Procedure:

1. Assemble all the ingredients at one place.
2. Wrap the ham around the asparagus stalks.
3. Eat as it is or may be steam for some time.

4. Use any dipping of your liking such as mayonnaise or béarnaise.

5. Smell the aroma and now you can serve.

Preparation time: 5 to 10 minutes

Cooking time: 10 to 15 minutes

Servings: 1 to 2

King sized Bacon and Egg Covered in Tomato Sauce

This recipe is going to sizzle your taste buds. Get the taste of this simple yet really tantalizing recipe.

What you need:

- 4 fresh sage leaves (Sliced)
- 4 medium Eggs
- 1 onion, finely chopped
- 1 turnip, diced
- 1 to 2 cup of parsley (Sliced)
- 4 strips of bacon (Diced)
- 2 to 3 cups of tomato passata
- 1 to 2 cup of chives (Sliced)
- 1 to 2 tablespoon Ghee

Procedure:

1. Gather all the items.

2. Place the turnip in a pan of boiling water and cook for around 5 to 10 minutes.

3. Please heat up a pan over medium heat and then you should add the onion and ghee. Start cooking and occasionally turn for around 5 to 10 minutes.

4. Now we can proceed to the next most important step.

5. Combine the bacon and cook until fried.

6. Now combine the ghee, tomato Passata, chives and sage leaves to the pan with the bacon.

7. Please crack the eggs on the top of sauce & cover it. Cook for around 10 to 15 minutes.

8. One thing remains to be done now.

9. Put the parsley on top.

10. Enjoy your Bacon and Egg covered in tomato sauce!

Servings: 2 to 3

Overall time to prepare: 30 to 40 minutes

Classic Paleo Bread

This is one of the simplest yet classic recipes.

What you need:

- 3 to 4 tbsp almond flour
- Salt
- ¼ cup ground golden flax
- 6 eggs (Pastured)
- ¾ coconut butter
- 2 to 3 tablespoons honey
- 1 to 2 tbsp baking soda
- ¼ cup olive oil (Melted)
- About 1/2 to 1 tsp apple cider vinegar

Procedure:

1. Gather all the items.
2. Preheat your oven to about 350 to 360° F.
3. Please line a 10 x 5" loaf pan with parchment.
4. Then grease it with little olive oil.
5. Now we can go ahead to the next most important step.
6. Blend the following ingredients in a blender: coconut butter, honey, eggs, olive oil and apple cider vinegar.
7. Now combine the following ingredients in another bowl: salt, baking soda, almond flour and the golden flax.
8. Mix the apple cider vinegar mixture with the golden flax mixture.

9. Now place it into the loaf pan and bake for around 40 to 50 minutes.

10. Now, only one main thing remains to be done now.

11. Let the bread cool down for around 10 to 15 minutes.

12. Enjoy your Classic Paleo Bread!

Servings: 4 to 5

Overall time to prepare: 60 to 70 minutes

Fantastic Egg Avocados

What you need:

- Pepper
- 2 to 3 tablespoons chives (Sliced)
- 4 to 5 avocados
- 8 to 9 medium eggs

Procedure:

1. Assemble all the ingredients at one place.
2. Preheat your oven to about 400 to 410° F.
3. Please slice the avocados in half & take out the pit.
4. Please scoop 2 to 3 tablespoons of avocado flesh from the middle of the avocado.

5. Now we can proceed to the next most important step.
6. Put the avocados in a baking dish.
7. Crack an egg in each avocado.
8. Place in the oven and bake for 20 to 25 minutes.
9. Now come to the most important steps.
10. Withdraw from the oven and place the chives and pepper on each avocado.
11. Enjoy your egg avocados!

Smell the aroma and serve.

Servings: 6 to 7

Overall time to prepare: 30 to 40 minutes

Historic Italian Paleo Eggs

This is one recipe that is tasty and can be prepared with ease if you follow the instructions carefully.

What you need:

- 1 cup of baby spinach (Shredded)
- ¼ almond milk
- ¼ pound sausage, crumbled and withdraw the casings
- 1 Roma tomato (Sliced)
- 4 eggs
- Salt & pepper
- 1/2 tsps tomato paste
- 1/4 to 1 teaspoon oregano (Dried)
- 1 to 2 tsp almond meal
- Olive oil

Procedure:

1. Assemble all the items at one place.
2. Preheat your oven to about 350 to 360° F.
3. Grease 4 small baking dishes.
4. Layer each baking dish with the spinach, crumbled sausage and tomatoes.
5. In a small bowl: whisk the almond meal & milk, salt, oregano, pepper and tomato paste.
6. Put the sauce in each baking dish.
7. Put the 4 baking dishes in the oven and bake for around 15 to 20 minutes.
8. Now please remove the baking dishes from the oven and

increase the oven to about 410 to 420° F.

9. Crack an egg in each baking dish. Do not brake the yolk.

10. One thing remains to be done now.

11. Bake for around 10 to 15 minutes.

12. Enjoy your Italian Paleo eggs!

Serves: 4 to 5

Total time to now prepare: 35 to 40 minutes

Simple Apple and Squash Soup

This recipe is simply amazing and it is not even hard in your pocket. So enjoy making this recipe.

What you need:

- Sage (1/2 to 1 tsp.)
- Apple (1 cored)
- Sea salt (1 pinch)
- Almond milk (2 cups unsweetened)
- Kombucha squash (1 skin removed)
- Powdered onion (1/2 to 1 teaspoon.)
- Garlic (2 cloves)

Procedure:

1. Gather all the items.

2. Now prepare the kombucha squash by cutting it in half vertically and place both side face down on top of a cooking sheet.
3. Ensure your oven has been preheated to about 410 to 420 degrees F.
4. One thing remains to be done now.
5. Cook the squash for 45 to 55 minutes.
6. Placed the cooked squash and the other items and blended thoroughly.
7. Smell the aroma and serve.

Speedy Apricot Power Bars

What you need:

- 2 to 3 tbsp vanilla extract
- 1/2 to 1 tsp sea salt
- 4 to 5 cups pecans
- 2 cups dried apricots
- 4 eggs

Procedure:

1. Assemble all the items.
2. In a processor grind the pecans and apricots until the texture is love gravel.
3. Combine vanilla extract, eggs and salt and blend again.
4. Put mixture in a greased baking dish.

5. Now please bake for 25 to 35 minutes in a preheated oven at about 350 to 360° F.

6. Smell the aroma and serve.

Awesome Baked White Fish

This is one of my secrets recipes. Chefs all over the world will not be happy on knowing that I shared this one with you.

What you need:

- Salt (as per taste)
- 2 to 3 tbsp grass-fed butter
- Pepper (as per taste)
- 4 white fish fillets (fish as per your choice)
- Zest of 1 to 2 lemon
- Juice of 1 to 2 lemon

Procedure:

1. Assemble all the items.
2. The oven should be preheated to about 340 to 360° F.
3. Take a baking dish and place 4 to 5 fillets of fish.

4. Place a skillet on medium flame. Melt the butter.
5. Now come to the next important step.
6. You should add the lemon juice and lemon zest. Top with few salt and black pepper (as per taste).
7. Now pour the butter mixture on the fish and pop it into the oven for 15 to 20 minutes or may be until the fish is done.
8. Enjoy!

Strong Breakfast Cinnamon Sweet Potatoes

What you need:

- 1 to 2 tbsp coconut oil
- 1 to 2 tsp cinnamon
- 1 to 2 tbsp honey
- 4 sweet potatoes, peeled and cubed
- Salt (as per taste)
- 1 to 2 teaspoon nutmeg

Procedure:

1. Assemble all the items at one place.
2. Boil/cook the sweet potato cubes. Once cooked, toss with the spices and salt.

3. Heat up the coconut oil in a large pan. Now you should add in the sweet potatoes.
4. One thing remains to be done now.
5. Sauté the mix for 5 to 10 minutes or until it turns golden brown.
6. Drizzle honey over the sweet potatoes.
7. Smell the aroma and then you can serve.

Simple Breakfast Sausage Patties

What you need:

- Black pepper (as per taste)
- 1 to 2 tablespoon minced garlic
- 1 to 2 tsp sage
- 2 to 3 tablespoon coconut oil
- 1 to 2 teaspoon paprika
- 1 to 2 tsp fennel seeds
- White pepper (as per taste)
- Pinch of salt
- 1 pound chicken, ground
- Cayenne pepper (as per taste)

Procedure:

1. Assemble all the ingredients at one place.
2. Blend chicken, garlic and all the spices in a bowl. Blend well. Form this mixture into 2-oz patties; you'll sizzle your taste

buds and get the taste of this simple yet really tantalizing recipe.

3. Now come to the most important step.

4. Melt half of the oil in a skillet and cook the patties for 5 to 10 minutes on both the sides or until golden brown – make sure the middle is no longer pink.

5. Now you can serve them hot with a sauce of your choice.

Easy Carrot Cake Cookies

You are lucky. Want to know why? I am sharing my amazing recipe with you people.

What you need:

- 2 cups coconut (Shredded)
- 6 carrots, peeled and shredded
- 5 to 6 eggs
- 3 to 4 tsp vanilla
- 3 cups almonds (Sliced)
- 1 to 2 tsp nutmeg (Grated)
- 1 to 2 tsp cinnamon
- 1 cup almonds meal
- 3 to 4 teaspoon coconut oil

Procedure:

1. Assemble all the items.

2. The oven should be preheated to about 340 to 360° F.
3. Grind almonds, carrots, cinnamon, vanilla, nutmeg, coconut and almond meal in a food processor.
4. One thing remains to be done now.
5. Pour in the oil and blend; now you should add the eggs and blend it again.
6. Drop even-sized cookies with a spoon or may be scoop onto a lined baking sheet. Bake for 25 to 30 minutes, till done.
7. Smell the aroma and serve.

Awesome Chicken and Mushroom Stew

What you need:

- 1 to 2 teaspoon paprika
- 2 bell peppers
- 1 to 2 tablespoon tapioca starch, dissolved in some cold water
- 6 minced cloves of garlic
- 1 to 2 onion
- Chicken cubes
- Coconut oil for cooking
- Salt (as per taste)
- Pepper (as per taste)
- 3 cups hot homemade chicken broth

Procedure:

1. Assemble all the items.
2. Now wash all of the vegetables, and then cut them well.

3. Sauté the vegetables in coconut oil.
4. Now we can go ahead to the next most important step.
5. Once done, set away in a bowl.
6. Now take the garlic in the pan and sauté with the chicken till the chicken becomes golden brown. Season with paprika, salt and pepper.
7. Combine the broth and let it simmer with the tapioca starch mixture.
8. One thing remains to be done now.
9. Cook till it thickens.
10. Now you can serve with the sautéed veggies on the side.

Mind Blowing Roasted Butternut Squash Salad

My friend invited me over for lunch and taught me this amazing recipe.

What you need:

- Salt (as per taste)
- 1 to 2 tablespoon oregano
- Freshly ground black pepper (as per taste)
- 2 to 3 lbs butternut squash, peeled and cubed
- 1 to 2 tbsp coconut oil
- 1 to 2 tablespoon smoked paprika

Procedure:

1. Assemble all the items.

2. Preheat the oven to about 400 to 410° F.
3. Flip the squash with the spices and oil until evenly coated; season with salt and pepper. Blend again.
4. Now come to the most important step.
5. Roast squash in the oven till it becomes soft and gets a brown crust.
6. Serve hot.
7. Enjoy.

Wonderful Pumpkin Pecan Pancakes

What you need:

- 1 to 2 tsp pumpkin pie spice
- 2 to 3 tbsp raw honey
- Melted butter or coconut oil for cooking pancakes
- 1/2 to 1 cup almond flour
- Pinch of cinnamon
- 2 to 3 tablespoon coconut flour
- ¼ teaspoon baking powder
- 1 to 2 tbsp roughly sliced pecans
- 1/2 to 1 cup pumpkin puree
- Pinch of salt
- ¾ cup egg whites

Procedure:

1. Assemble all the items at one place.

2. Combine dry items in one bowl.

3. Whisk the wet items (puree, honey and eggs) in the different bowl and combine this mixture to the bowl of dry items.

4. Now we can go ahead to the next most important step.

5. Heat up a griddle over medium heat and melt butter or may be oil on it.

6. Pour the batter (the approximately ¼ cup at a time) on the griddle and spread out to make a pancake.

7. Please cook for 3 to 5 minutes on one side, toss above and cook for 5 to 10 minutes on the other side.

8. Only one more thing remains now.

9. Repeat with left batter.

10.	Now you can serve hot.

11.	Smell the aroma and serve.

Stunning Sashimi Salad

This is one of the rarest recipes. Keep it secret.

What you need:

- 4 handfuls kale leaves
- 2 to 3 Alfonso mangoes, peeled and sliced
- 1 to 2 tablespoon honey
- 6 to 7 tbsp tamari sauce
- 2 to 3 teaspoon vinegar
- 4 to 5 tablespoon olive oil
- 1 to 2 pound salmon sashimi, sliced finely

Procedure:

1. Assemble all the ingredients at one place.

2. In a bowl you should add olive oil, tamari sauce, honey and vinegar to make the dressing.
3. One thing remains to be done now.
4. Add the kale leaves.
5. Plate the salad and add salmon and mangoes.
6. Enjoy!!

This is the king recipe out there. There are no words to express this recipe.

Supreme Tuna Salad

This recipe is quick and amazing. You will love it.

What you need:

- Salt (as per taste)
- 1 stalk celery (Shredded)
- 1 to 2 English cucumber (Shredded)
- Zest of 1/2 lemon
- 1 fresh green onion, finely sliced
- Juice of 1/2 lemon
- 2 to 3 tbsp Paleo mayonnaise
- Freshly ground black pepper (as per taste)
- 2 to 3 large tomatoes (Sliced)

- 6 oz wild albacore tuna, pre-cooked

Procedure:

1. Assemble all the items.
2. Mix the onions, celery, lemon juice mayonnaise, and lemon zest in a bowl. Season with salt and pepper.
3. Combine the tomatoes, tuna and cucumber; toss well to blend. Now serve at once or chill and now you can serve later.
4. Smell the aroma and now you can serve.

Insane Beef, Spinach and Avocado Salad

What you need:

- Salt, to taste
- 1 avocado, peeled and sliced
- 8 to 9 oz quality roast beef, thinly sliced
- 2 tomatoes, thinly sliced
- 3 cups baby spinach
- About 2 to 3 tablespoon extra virgin olive oil
- 1 large red onion, sliced & separated into rings

For the dressing:

- 1 to 2 tbsp mustard
- 1 to 2 tablespoon extra virgin olive oil
- 2 to 3 tbsp lemon juice

Procedure:

1. Assemble all the items.
2. Mix all dressing items in a deep bowl and stir until smooth.
3. Heat up olive oil in a large skillet and with care sauté the onions and beef. Start cooking the beef is heated through.
4. Now come to the most important part.
5. Toss together the beef, spinach, tomatoes and avocado in a large salad bowl.
6. Now season with salt you have, drizzle with the dressing and serve.
7. Enjoy!!

Serves 4 to 6

Prep time: 5 to 10 minutes

Magical Grilled Chicken Salad

Have this magical recipe. It will make your day!!

What you need:

- 1 to 2 tbsp balsamic vinegar
- 1/3 cup black olives (Pitted)
- Salt and black pepper, to taste
- 1 red bell pepper (Sliced)
- 2 to 3 cups grilled chicken breasts (Diced)
- 3 to 4 green onions (Sliced)
- 1 cup grape tomatoes
- 1 to 2 teaspoon dried oregano
- 2 to 3 tbsp extra virgin olive oil

Procedure:

1. Assemble all the ingredients at one place.

2. Put chicken in a deep salad bowl. Combine in the grape tomatoes, onion, red pepper and olives. Season with salt and pepper.
3. Flip lightly to combine, top with oregano, balsamic vinegar and olive oil, and serve.
4. Enjoy!!

Serves: 4 to 5

Prep time: 10 to 15 minutes

Mouth Watering Banana-Berry Pancakes

What you need:

- 2 to 3 tbsp almond butter
- ¼ to 1 tsp cinnamon
- ⅓ cup raspberries (Mashed)
- 6 to 7 egg whites, lightly beaten
- 2 bananas (Mashed)

Procedure:

1. Assemble all the items at one place.
2. Please spray skillet or griddle with a cooking spray. In a large or medium bowl, blend the bananas, raspberries, egg whites and almond butter until smooth.

3. Please pour the batter into skillet using ½ to 1 cup for every pancake.
4. Now please wait for 5 to 10 minutes before flipping.
5. One thing remains to be done now.
6. Pancakes. Please cook for an additional 3 to 5 minutes or so till golden brown.
7. Please serve with a topping of cinnamon or may be fresh fruit.
8. Enjoy!!

Servings 2 to 4

Tempting Egg Salad Lettuce Wraps

What you need:

- 2 to 3 large lettuce leaves, such as iceberg or romaine, intact and un-torn
- Lemon juice, for seasoning
- 2 to 3 tablespoons relish or chopped pickles
- 2 to 3 large hard-boiled eggs, peeled and chopped
- Freshly ground black pepper, to taste
- 2 to 3 tbsps olive-oil mayonnaise

Procedure:

1. Assemble all the items at one place.

2. Put sliced eggs, mayo, and relish in a bowl and mix thoroughly to combine. Season with freshly ground black pepper.
3. Now come to the next important step.
4. Please divide egg salad mixture evenly among the lettuces leaves & wrap, but not tightly, as you don't want the leaves to tear.
5. Please season with lemon juice if desired.
6. Now serve immediately with baby carrots for a healthy and filling lunch.
7. Smell the aroma and serve.

Serves 2 to 4

Interesting High-Protein Frittata

What you need:

- 8 to 9 large eggs
- 1/2 small onion (Chopped)
- 4 to 5 strips of uncured, nitrate-free bacon, cooked and crumbled
- 1 to 2 tablespoon olive or coconut oil
- 2 to 3 cups baby spinach leaves
- ½ to 1 cup mushrooms (Sliced)
- Freshly ground black pepper, to taste

Procedure:

1. Gather all the items.
2. Preheat oven to about 350 to 360 degrees F.

3. Heat a large ovenproof skillet over medium heat and add the oil and vegetables.
4. Sauté until tender.
5. Remove from skillet and set aside.
6. Please beat the eggs in a large or medium bowl & add the cooked vegetables.
7. Season with freshly ground black pepper.
8. Now pour mixture into the skillet and place in the oven.
9. Only one more thing remains to be done now.
10. Please bake for 10 to 15 minutes or till eggs are firm to the touch.
11. Top with crumbled bacon and serve immediately.
12. Enjoy!

Servings 4 to 6

Powerful Paleo Granola

Learn this one by heart and make it for your friends and family. They will love it.

What you need:

- 1/3 cup raw pumpkin seeds
- 1 to 2 cup raw sunflower seeds
- 1 to 2 cup raisins
- 1 cup raw pecans
- 1 cup raw sliced almonds
- 1 cup raw walnuts
- 1 cup unsweetened coconut (Shredded)
- 1 cup Medjool dates (Shredded)

Procedure:

1. Assemble all the items.
2. Now please soak nuts & seeds overnight in warm water, approximately 10 to 12 hours.
3. Drain well.
4. Now we can proceed to the next most important step.
5. Then spread the nuts and seeds on a baking sheet in an even layer.
6. Set oven to the lowest temperature possible and place the baking sheet in the oven door open, dehydrate nuts for 12 hours.
7. Allow cooling.
8. Chop nuts and seeds and blend with the coconut, dates, and raisins.

9. Now you can serve either as a snack or may be with unsweetened almond milk as a breakfast cereal.

10.   Smell the aroma and serve.

Servings 8 to 9

Crazy Paleo Spinach Quiche

What you need:

- ½ to 1 teaspoon ground nutmeg
- 1 cup chopped fresh spinach
- ½ to 1 cup plain almond milk
- ½ to 1 tsp salt
- 1 to 2 tsp olive oil, plus more for greasing the pan
- ½ to 1 tsp freshly ground black pepper
- 1/2 cup sliced red onion
- 8 to 9 large eggs (Beaten)

Procedure:

1. Assemble all the ingredients at one place.

2. Preheat oven to about 350 to 360 degrees F.

3. Grease a 9-inch glass pie plate.

4. In a small skillet, heat up the olive oil over medium heat, and sauté the spinach, salt, pepper, onion, and nutmeg for about 5 to 10 minutes, or may be just until the onions are translucent.

5. Now we can go ahead to the next most important step.

6. Stir the eggs and almond milk together in a small bowl. Combine the spinach mixture, whisk, and now pour into the pie plate.

7. One thing remains to be done now.

8. Bake the quiche on the middle oven rack for 30 to 40 minutes,

or until the middle is properly set.

9. Now you can serve warm or may be at room temperature.

Smell the aroma and now you can serve.

Serves 4 to 5

Cool Poached Eggs and Root Vegetable Hash

What you need:

- Freshly ground black pepper, to taste
- 4 to 5 large eggs
- 1 small onion (Shredded)
- 2 to 3 tablespoons olive or may be coconut oil
- 1/3 large beet, peeled and sliced
- 1 fresh rosemary, finely sliced
- 1 to 2 medium turnip, peeled and sliced
- 1 to 2 clove garlic (minced)

Procedure:

1. Assemble all the items at one place.

2. Preheat oven to about 400 to 410 degrees F. Flip veggies in the oil and lay on a single-layer sheet pan. Sprinkle on shredded rosemary. Season with freshly ground black pepper.

3. Please roast for about 10 to 15 minutes or so, and then remove from oven, and add garlic.

4. Please roast for 10 more minutes, or may be until crispy around the edges.

5. One thing remains to be done now.

6. While the veggies are cooking, poach eggs in a pot of simmering water, till just cooked.

7. To serve, divide the root vegetables between 2 plates and

top with 2 eggs. Serve
immediately.
8. Enjoy!

Serves 2 to 4

Thanks for reading my book.

www.ingramcontent.com/pod-product-compliance
Lightning Source LLC
Chambersburg PA
CBHW070825240726

48654CB00007B/482